Nutritionist's Ninja Creami Protein Cookbook Recipes 2025

Tasty, Guilt-Free Recipes with Nutritious Ingredients

Clara Winslow

DISCLAIMER

This information is for your personal use ONLY. You cannot distribute, copy, reproduce, or otherwise sell this product or information in any form whatsoever, including but not limited to: electronic, or mechanical, including photocopying, recording, or by any informational storage or retrieval system without expressed written, dated and signed permission from the author. All copyrights are reserved.

The information, including but not limited to, text, graphics, images and other material contained in this guide are for informational purposes only. No material from this guide is intended to be a substitute for professional medical advice, diagnosis or treatment.

Always seek the advice of your physician or other qualified health care provider with any questions you may have regarding a medical condition or treatment and before undertaking a new health care regimen, and never disregard professional medical advice or delay in seeking it because of something you have read in this guide.

Table of CONTENTS

INTRODUCTION

Welcome to the Ninja Creami Protein Cookbook!

I'm excited to guide you on this flavorful journey toward creating delicious, protein-rich frozen treats that are not only satisfying but also nutritious.

In today's health-conscious world, finding desserts that align with your dietary goals can be challenging. This cookbook is designed to inspire you to make indulgent yet guilt-free treats right at home, using the versatile Ninja Creami.

With a variety of recipes that cater to different tastes and dietary preferences, you'll discover how easy it is to enjoy homemade desserts without compromising your health

Clara Winslow's Story

I'm Clara Winslow, a certified nutritionist, and I'm thrilled to share my passion for healthy cooking with you.

My journey into the world of nutrition began in my childhood kitchen, where I learned the joys of cooking and the importance of wholesome ingredients. Growing up, I was always surrounded by the delightful aroma of home-cooked meals, and it ignited a lifelong love for creating nutritious yet delicious dishes.

After earning my Bachelor's degree in Nutritional Science, I dedicated my career to helping families navigate their dietary needs, ensuring they can enjoy flavorful meals that support their health.

HOW TO BEST USE THIS *Cookbook*

This cookbook is structured to be user-friendly and accessible for cooks of all skill levels. You'll find a variety of recipes categorized by type, including smoothies, ice creams, and frozen treats.

Each recipe includes a list of ingredients, step-by-step instructions, and a detailed nutritional breakdown, allowing you to make informed choices about what you're consuming.

Whether you're looking for a post-workout protein boost or a sweet treat to enjoy with your family, this book has something for everyone.

Why Clara Winslow is an Authority on Protein and the Ninja Creami

As a certified nutritionist, I understand the vital role protein plays in our diets. It is essential for muscle repair, immune function, and overall health. The Ninja Creami is a fantastic tool for incorporating high-protein ingredients into your dessert repertoire, transforming everyday ingredients into delicious frozen treats. My expertise allows me to provide you with recipes that not only taste incredible but also help you meet your protein needs.

Clara's Background in Nutritional Science

With a Bachelor's degree in Nutritional Science, I have spent years working in various healthcare settings, helping clients understand their dietary needs and make healthier choices. My experience has taught me the importance of balance—enjoying the foods we love while also prioritizing our health. This philosophy is woven throughout the recipes in this cookbook.

Experience in Developing High-Protein Recipes

Throughout my career, I have dedicated myself to creating high-protein recipes that are both enjoyable and easy to prepare. This cookbook features a wide array of treats that incorporate protein-rich ingredients, such as protein powders, Greek yogurt, and nut butters. Each recipe has been carefully crafted to ensure you can indulge in delicious desserts while effectively meeting your nutritional goals.

Passion for Healthy Eating and Family Nutrition

At the heart of my work is a genuine passion for healthy eating and family nutrition. I believe that food should not only nourish our bodies but also bring joy and connection to our lives. My goal with this cookbook is to inspire families to come together in the kitchen, creating memories while enjoying nutritious treats that everyone can enjoy.

Thank you for joining me on this exciting culinary adventure! Let's dive into the world of protein-rich frozen treats and discover how the Ninja Creami can help you create delicious desserts that promote health and happiness!

Understanding THE NINJA CREAMI

Why the *Ninja Creami?*

The Ninja Creami is a revolutionary kitchen appliance designed for creating a variety of frozen treats, including ice creams, sorbets, and smoothie bowls, with incredible ease. This innovative machine allows you to turn your favorite ingredients into creamy, delicious desserts in just minutes.

With its powerful processing capabilities, the Ninja Creami takes the hassle out of making homemade frozen treats, giving you the freedom to experiment with flavors and textures while ensuring that your creations are both enjoyable and nutritious.

Benefits of Using the Ninja Creami for Protein-Rich Recipes

When it comes to incorporating protein into your diet, the Ninja Creami excels at making healthy frozen treats that satisfy your cravings without sacrificing nutrition. Here are some key benefits of using this appliance for protein-rich recipes:

1. **Enhanced Nutritional Value:** The Ninja Creami allows you to easily integrate protein-rich ingredients such as protein powder, Greek yogurt, and nut butters into your desserts. This means you can enjoy sweet treats while meeting your protein intake goals, which is particularly beneficial for active individuals and families.
2. **Versatile Recipe Options:** With the ability to create a wide range of frozen desserts, the Ninja Creami enables you to experiment with various flavor combinations and ingredients. Whether you're in the mood for a rich chocolate ice cream or a fruity sorbet, you can easily adapt recipes to include protein sources, making it suitable for different dietary preferences.
3. **Time-Saving Convenience:** The Ninja Creami streamlines the process of making frozen treats. You can prepare your protein-packed bases in advance, freeze them, and then process them quickly when you're ready to enjoy a delicious dessert. This makes it easier to fit healthy eating into your busy lifestyle.
4. **Control Over Ingredients:** By making frozen treats at home, you have complete control over the ingredients you use. This means you can avoid artificial additives, excessive sugars, and unhealthy fats commonly found in store-bought options. The Ninja Creami empowers you to create desserts that are not only delicious but also align with your health goals.

Getting Started

Key Features and Functions

To make the most of your Ninja Creami experience, it's important to familiarize yourself with its key features and functions:

1. **Processing Functions:** The Ninja Creami comes equipped with several functions tailored for different types of frozen treats:
   - **Ice Cream Function:** Perfect for creamy ice creams, this function processes your frozen base to achieve the ideal consistency while incorporating protein-rich ingredients.
   - **Sorbet Function:** Designed for making refreshing sorbets, this setting ensures your fruity bases are smooth and icy without becoming overly hard.
   - **Gelato Function:** This function produces denser and creamier results, ideal for rich desserts that require a velvety texture.
   - **Mix-In Function:** After processing your base, this function allows you to fold in mix-ins like chocolate chips or nuts without over-processing, ensuring a delightful textural contrast.
2. **User-Friendly Control Panel:** The intuitive control panel features easy-to-use buttons for each processing function, along with a digital display that guides you through the process. This makes operating the Ninja Creami simple, even for those who are new to making frozen treats.
3. **Compact and Stylish Design:** The Ninja Creami's sleek design fits seamlessly into any kitchen. Its compact size means it won't take up too much counter space, and its modern appearance adds a touch of style to your culinary space.
4. **Easy Cleanup:** All removable parts, including the pint containers and lids, are dishwasher safe, ensuring that cleaning up after your culinary adventures is quick and hassle-free. The base of the machine can be wiped down with a damp cloth to keep it clean and ready for your next creation.

Healthy PROTEIN SOURCES

Essential Ingredients for
High-Protein Recipes

Incorporating high-protein ingredients into your meals and snacks is essential for maintaining energy levels, supporting muscle recovery, and promoting overall health. Here are some key ingredients to consider when crafting your protein-rich recipes in The Nutritionist Ninja Creami Cookbook:

1. **Protein Powder:** A convenient and versatile way to boost protein intake, protein powders can be added to smoothies, ice creams, and baked goods. Choose high-quality options, such as whey protein, pea protein, or hemp protein, to suit your dietary preferences.
2. **Greek Yogurt:** Greek yogurt is an excellent source of protein and adds creaminess to your frozen desserts. It's also rich in probiotics, which are beneficial for gut health. Opt for plain varieties to avoid added sugars.
3. **Cottage Cheese:** Cottage cheese is packed with protein and can be used in smoothies or blended into ice creams for added creaminess. It has a mild flavor that pairs well with both sweet and savory dishes.
4. **Nut Butters:** Nut butters, such as almond butter or peanut butter, not only provide protein but also healthy fats. They can add richness and flavor to shakes, ice creams, and energy bites.
5. **Chia Seeds:** Chia seeds are a great source of protein, fiber, and omega-3 fatty acids. They absorb liquid and create a gel-like texture, making them perfect for puddings and smoothies.
6. **Silken Tofu:** Silken tofu is an excellent dairy-free source of protein that can be blended into smoothies or ice creams for a smooth, creamy texture. It's also versatile and can be used in both sweet and savory dishes.
7. **Egg Whites:** For those who consume eggs, egg whites are a high-protein ingredient that can be incorporated into various recipes, adding fluffiness and nutrition.

Tips for Choosing *Healthy Substitutes*

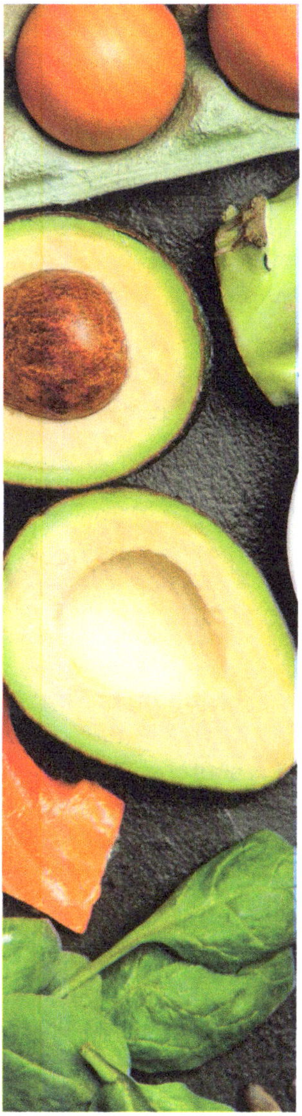

Opt for Whole Foods: Focus on using whole, minimally processed ingredients. Fresh fruits, vegetables, nuts, seeds, and whole grains provide essential nutrients and are generally healthier options compared to processed alternatives.

Read Labels: When purchasing packaged ingredients, such as protein powders or nut butters, check the labels for added sugars, preservatives, and artificial ingredients. Look for products with minimal ingredients that align with your health goals.

Prioritize Nutrient Density: Choose ingredients that offer a high amount of nutrients relative to their calorie content. For instance, berries provide antioxidants and vitamins while being low in calories, making them an excellent addition to your recipes.

Consider Dietary Preferences: Be mindful of dietary restrictions and preferences when selecting ingredients. Many recipes can easily be adapted to be vegan, gluten-free, or nut-free by swapping in suitable alternatives.

Nutritional Considerations for Protein Intake

Daily Protein Needs

The recommended daily protein intake varies based on age, activity level, and health goals. As a general guideline, adults should aim for about 0.8 grams of protein per kilogram of body weight. Athletes or those engaged in intense physical activity may require more.

Distributing Protein Intake

It's beneficial to spread your protein intake throughout the day across meals and snacks. Incorporating high-protein treats like those in this cookbook can help you reach your daily goals without feeling overwhelmed.

Balancing Macronutrients

While protein is essential, it's important to maintain a balanced diet that includes carbohydrates and healthy fats. This ensures that your body has the necessary fuel for energy and overall health.

Listening to Your Body

Pay attention to how your body responds to different protein sources. Some individuals may find certain proteins easier to digest than others. Experimenting with various ingredients can help you identify what works best for you.

By integrating these healthy protein sources into your recipes and following these guidelines, you can create delicious frozen treats that align with your nutritional goals. Let's dive into the recipes that will help you unleash your creativity in the kitchen while maintaining a focus on health!

Protein Packed
SMOOTHIES & SHAKES

Chocolate Peanut Butter Protein Shake

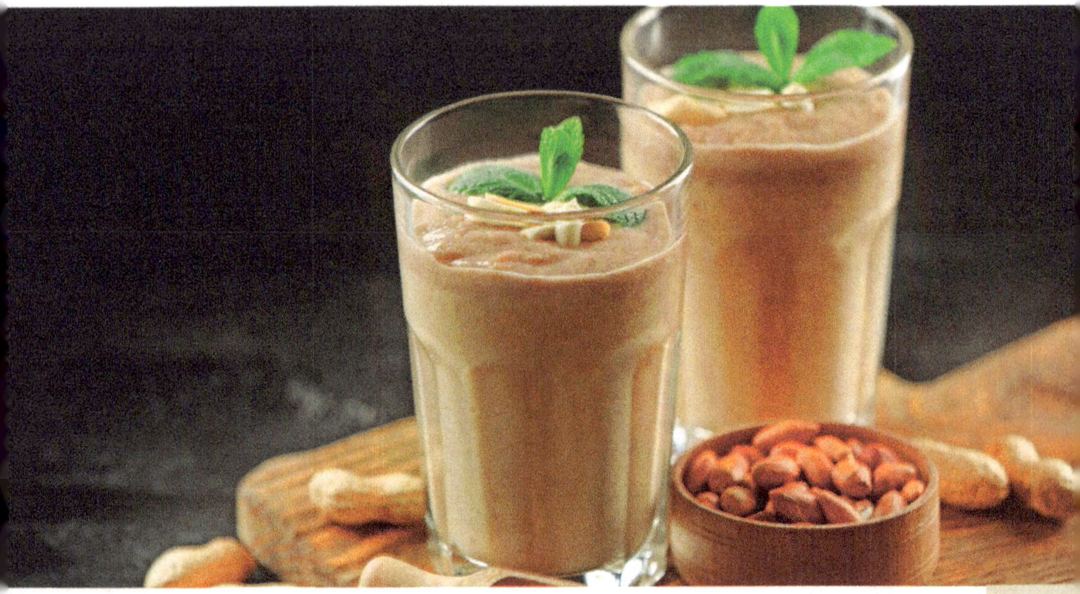

This Chocolate Peanut Butter Protein Shake is one of my go-to recipes for a quick and nutritious breakfast or a post-workout snack. Packed with protein from the chocolate protein powder and healthy fats from the peanut butter, it provides a satisfying and energizing boost to kick-start your day or refuel after exercise. I love the creamy texture and rich flavor, thanks to the combination of bananas and cocoa powder. This shake is not only delicious but also incredibly easy to make, making it a perfect choice for busy mornings or when you need a quick pick-me-up. I often whip this up for my family, and it's a hit with both my daughter, Emma, and my husband!

Ingredients

- 1 cup unsweetened almond milk (or any milk of choice)
- 1 scoop chocolate protein powder (whey or plant-based)
- 2 tablespoons natural peanut butter (or almond butter)
- 1 medium banana (fresh or frozen)
- 1 tablespoon cocoa powder (unsweetened)
- 1 teaspoon honey or maple syrup (optional, adjust to taste)
- A pinch of salt
- Ice cubes (optional, for a thicker texture)

Nutrition

Calories	**350**
Protein	**25 g**
Carbohydrates	**35 g**
Sugars	**15 g**
Fats (Total)	**15 g**
Saturated	**3 g**
Unsaturated	**12 g**
Fiber	**4 g**

Instructions

1. **Combine Ingredients:** In a blender, add the almond milk, chocolate protein powder, peanut butter, banana, cocoa powder, honey (if using), and a pinch of salt.
2. **Blend Until Smooth:** Blend on high speed until the mixture is completely smooth and creamy. If you prefer a thicker shake, add a few ice cubes and blend again until well combined.
3. **Taste and Adjust:** Taste the shake and adjust sweetness if needed by adding more honey or maple syrup. Blend again if you make any adjustments.
4. **Serve:** Pour the shake into a glass and enjoy immediately. You can also garnish with a sprinkle of cocoa powder or a few chocolate chips on top for an extra treat.

Nutritionist Tips

- **Protein Powder:** Choose a high-quality protein powder that fits your dietary needs. The flavor of the protein powder can influence the overall taste of the shake, so feel free to experiment with different brands and flavors.
- **Nut Butter Alternatives:** If you have nut allergies, consider using sunflower seed butter or tahini as a substitute for peanut butter.
- **Add-Ins:** For additional nutrition, you can blend in a handful of spinach or kale for extra vitamins and minerals without altering the flavor significantly.

Berry Blast Protein Smoothie

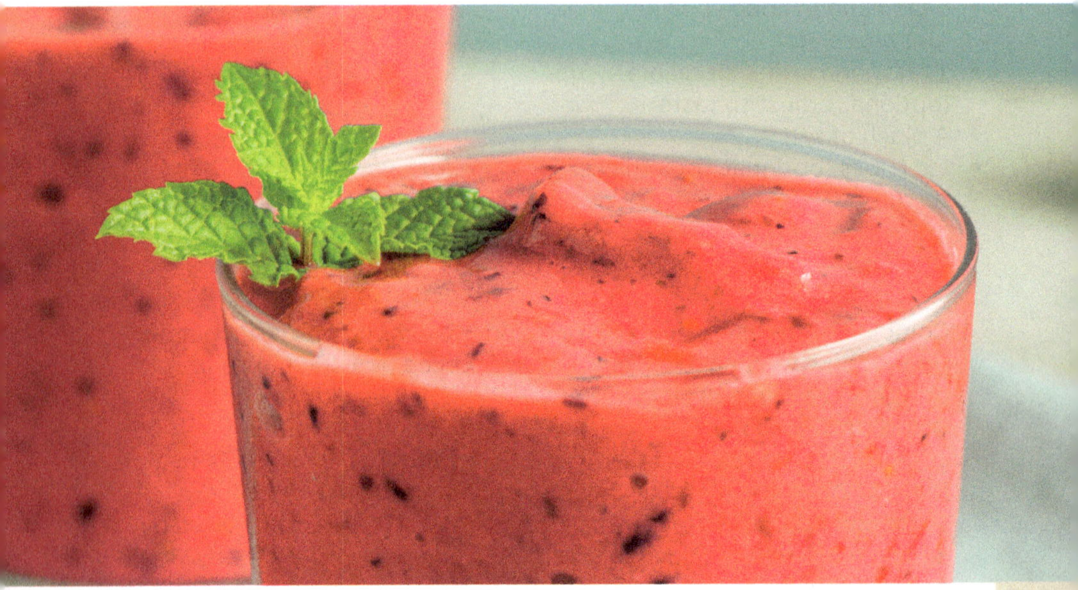

The Berry Blast Protein Smoothie is a vibrant and refreshing option that I often turn to for a quick breakfast or a revitalizing snack. Bursting with the natural sweetness of mixed berries, this smoothie not only satisfies your taste buds but also packs a powerful nutritional punch. Berries are rich in antioxidants, vitamins, and fiber, making them an excellent choice for promoting overall health. By adding protein powder and a splash of almond milk, you create a deliciously creamy texture while ensuring you're getting the protein you need to keep you energized throughout the day. This recipe is perfect for busy mornings or post-workout refueling, and it's an easy way to incorporate more fruits into your diet!

Ingredients

- 1 cup mixed berries (fresh or frozen; strawberries, blueberries, raspberries, blackberries)
- 1 cup unsweetened almond milk (or any milk of choice)
- 1 scoop vanilla protein powder (whey or plant-based)
- 1 banana (fresh or frozen)
- 1 tablespoon chia seeds (optional, for added fiber)
- 1 teaspoon honey or maple syrup (optional, adjust to taste)
- Ice cubes (optional, for a thicker texture)

Nutrition

Calories	**250**
Protein	**20 g**
Carbohydrates	**35 g**
Sugars	**15 g**
Fats (Total)	**5 g**
Saturated	**0.5 g**
Unsaturated	**4.5 g**
Fiber	**7 g**

Instructions

1. **Combine Ingredients:** In a blender, add the mixed berries, almond milk, protein powder, banana, chia seeds (if using), honey (if desired), and a handful of ice cubes.
2. **Blend Until Smooth:** Blend on high speed until the mixture is completely smooth and creamy. Adjust the thickness by adding more almond milk if needed, or add more ice for a thicker consistency.
3. **Taste and Adjust:** Taste the smoothie and adjust sweetness if necessary by adding more honey or maple syrup. Blend again if you make any adjustments.
4. **Serve:** Pour the smoothie into a glass and enjoy immediately. You can also garnish with additional berries or a sprinkle of chia seeds on top for an extra touch.

Nutritionist Tips

- **Choosing Berries:** Opt for a variety of berries to maximize the nutritional benefits. Fresh berries are fantastic, but frozen options work well too and can help create a thicker smoothie.
- **Protein Powder:** Select a protein powder that suits your dietary preferences. Vanilla flavor complements the berries beautifully, but feel free to experiment with other flavors.
- **Chia Seeds:** Adding chia seeds is a great way to boost the fiber content and provide healthy omega-3 fatty acids. They also help thicken the smoothie.

Tropical Protein Shake

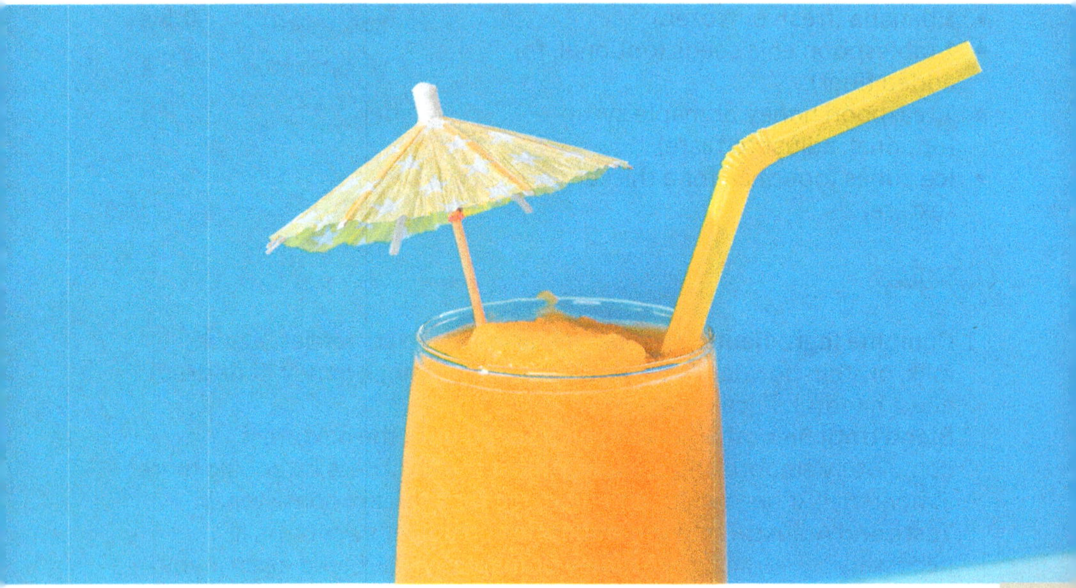

The Tropical Protein Shake is a delightful escape to paradise in a glass! Bursting with the vibrant flavors of tropical fruits like pineapple and mango, this shake is not only refreshing but also loaded with nutrients. The addition of protein powder makes it a great option for a post-workout recovery or a satisfying breakfast that keeps you energized throughout the day. I love whipping up this shake for my family during the warmer months, as it's a fantastic way to hydrate and enjoy the sweet taste of summer all year round. It's simple to prepare, and the bright, sunny flavors are sure to bring a smile to your face!

Ingredients

- 1 cup unsweetened coconut milk (or any milk of choice)
- 1 scoop vanilla protein powder (whey or plant-based)
- 1/2 cup frozen pineapple chunks
- 1/2 cup frozen mango chunks
- 1 medium banana (fresh or frozen)
- 1 tablespoon shredded coconut (unsweetened, optional)
- Ice cubes (optional, for a thicker texture)

Nutrition

Calories	**300**
Protein	**25 g**
Carbohydrates	**40 g**
Sugars	**18 g**
Fats (Total)	**7 g**
Saturated	**5 g**
Unsaturated	**2 g**
Fiber	**4 g**

Instructions

1. **Combine Ingredients:** In a blender, add the coconut milk, protein powder, frozen pineapple, frozen mango, banana, and shredded coconut (if using). If you prefer a thicker shake, add a handful of ice cubes.
2. **Blend Until Smooth:** Blend on high speed until the mixture is completely smooth and creamy. If the shake is too thick for your liking, you can add a little more coconut milk to achieve your desired consistency.
3. **Taste and Adjust:** Taste the shake and adjust sweetness if necessary by adding a bit of honey or maple syrup if you prefer. Blend again if you make any adjustments.
4. **Serve:** Pour the shake into a glass and enjoy immediately. For an extra tropical touch, garnish with a slice of fresh pineapple or a sprinkle of shredded coconut on top.

Nutritionist Tips

- **Fruit Selection:** Using frozen fruits not only adds a refreshing chill to your shake but also helps achieve a thicker texture. Fresh fruits work well too, but you may need to add more ice.
- **Coconut Milk Variations:** If you enjoy a stronger coconut flavor, use coconut cream instead of coconut milk. Just be mindful of the added calories and adjust the serving size accordingly.
- **Customization:** This shake is versatile; you can add spinach or kale for extra nutrients, or swap in different fruits like papaya or kiwi for a unique twist.

Guilt-Free
ICE CREAMS & FROZEN TREATS

Vanilla Protein Ice Cream

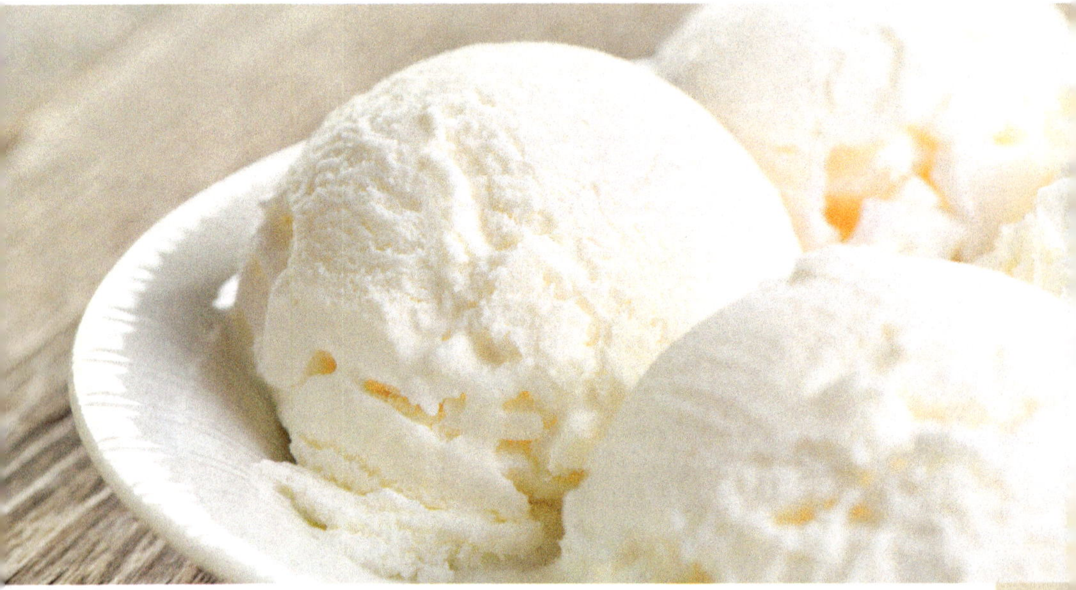

The Vanilla Protein Ice Cream is a staple recipe in my home, especially when I want to indulge my sweet tooth without the guilt. This creamy, rich ice cream is packed with protein, making it a fantastic option for a post-workout treat or a healthy dessert option after dinner. The simplicity of vanilla allows you to enjoy the pure flavor while also serving as a base for endless customization. I love to pair it with fresh fruits, nuts, or even a drizzle of homemade chocolate sauce. This recipe is not only easy to prepare but also perfect for satisfying cravings while keeping your nutritional goals in check!

Ingredients

- 2 cups unsweetened almond milk (or any milk of choice)
- 1 cup plain Greek yogurt (non-fat or full-fat based on preference)
- 1/2 cup vanilla protein powder (whey or plant-based)
- 1/4 cup honey or maple syrup (adjust to taste; can use sugar-free sweetener for lower sugar)
- 1 teaspoon pure vanilla extract
- Pinch of salt

Nutrition

Calories	**180**
Protein	**15 g**
Carbohydrates	**18 g**
Sugars	**7 g**
Fats (Total)	**6 g**
Saturated	**3 g**
Unsaturated	**3 g**
Fiber	**1 g**

Instructions

1. **Combine Ingredients:** In a mixing bowl, whisk together the almond milk, Greek yogurt, vanilla protein powder, honey (or sweetener), vanilla extract, and a pinch of salt until smooth and well combined.
2. **Cool the Mixture:** Chill the mixture in the refrigerator for about 30 minutes to ensure it's cold before freezing.
3. **Freeze the Base:** Pour the chilled mixture into your Ninja Creami pint container. Ensure it's filled to the fill line and then freeze for at least 24 hours.

Creami Processing

1. **Creami Processing:** After freezing, remove the pint from the freezer. Place it in your Ninja Creami machine, select the "Ice Cream" function, and process until smooth and creamy.
2. **Serve or Store:** Enjoy immediately for a soft-serve texture or return to the freezer for a firmer consistency. You can also customize by adding mix-ins like chocolate chips, nuts, or fresh fruit after processing.

Nutritionist Tips

- **Sweetener Options:** If you prefer a low-sugar option, consider using a sugar-free sweetener like erythritol or stevia. Adjust the amount based on your taste preference.
- **Texture Enhancement:** For an even creamier texture, consider adding a tablespoon of coconut cream or a small amount of nut butter to the mixture before freezing.
- **Mix-In Ideas:** This ice cream serves as a fantastic base for various mix-ins. Get creative by adding crushed cookies, fresh berries, or even a swirl of caramel or chocolate sauce after processing.

Chocolate Almond Protein Ice Cream

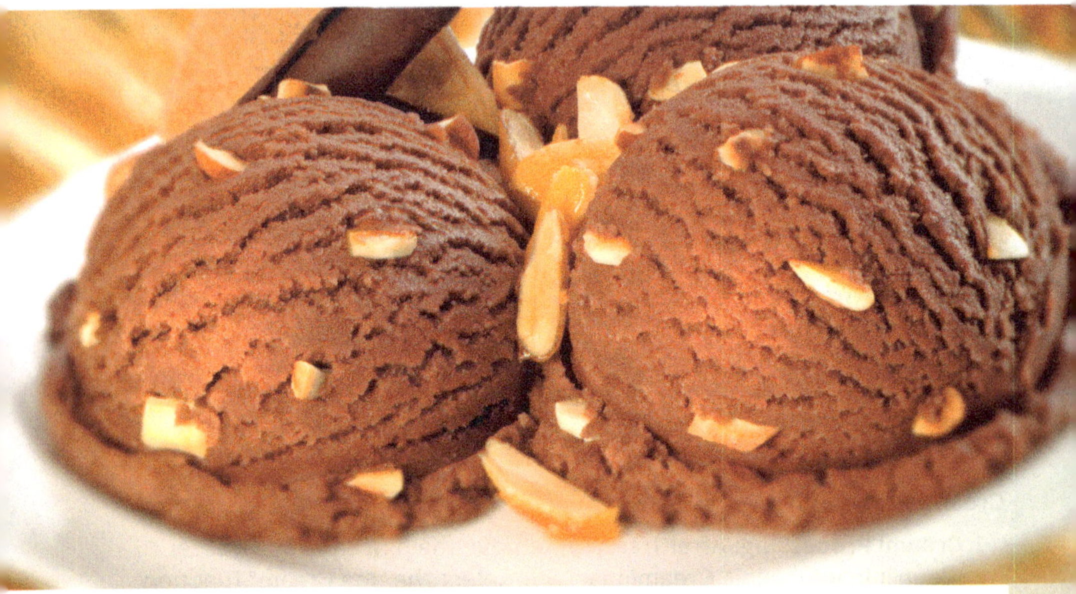

The Chocolate Almond Protein Ice Cream is a deliciously indulgent treat that combines the rich flavor of chocolate with the nutty goodness of almonds. As a certified nutritionist, I appreciate how this recipe provides a satisfying dessert that also supports your protein intake. With wholesome ingredients and the added benefits of protein powder, this ice cream is perfect for a post-workout recovery or a healthy treat any time of day. I often whip up this recipe when I want something sweet yet nutritious, and it never fails to impress my family and friends!

Ingredients

- 2 cups unsweetened almond milk (or any milk of choice)
- 1 cup plain Greek yogurt (non-fat or full-fat based on preference)
- 1/2 cup chocolate protein powder (whey or plant-based)
- 1/4 cup almond butter (or any nut butter)
- 1/4 cup maple syrup or honey (adjust to taste; can use sugar-free sweetener for lower sugar)
- 1 teaspoon pure vanilla extract
- 1/4 teaspoon almond extract (optional, for enhanced almond flavor)
- Pinch of salt

Nutrition

Calories	**250**
Protein	**20 g**
Carbohydrates	**22 g**
Sugars	**10 g**
Fats (Total)	**14 g**
Saturated	**3 g**
Unsaturated	**11 g**
Fiber	**3 g**

Instructions

1. **Combine Ingredients:** In a mixing bowl, whisk together the almond milk, Greek yogurt, chocolate protein powder, almond butter, maple syrup (or honey), vanilla extract, almond extract (if using), and a pinch of salt until smooth and well combined.
2. **Cool the Mixture:** Chill the mixture in the refrigerator for about 30 minutes to ensure it's cold before freezing.
3. **Freeze the Base:** Pour the chilled mixture into your Ninja Creami pint container. Ensure it's filled to the fill line and then freeze for at least 24 hours.

Creami Processing

1. **Creami Processing:** After freezing, remove the pint from the freezer. Place it in your Ninja Creami machine, select the "Ice Cream" function, and process until smooth and creamy.
2. **Serve or Store:** Enjoy immediately for a soft-serve texture or return to the freezer for a firmer consistency. For added texture, consider folding in some chopped almonds or chocolate chips after processing.

Nutritionist Tips

- **Mix-In Ideas:** This ice cream pairs wonderfully with various mix-ins, such as chopped dark chocolate, crushed cookies, or additional nuts. Get creative and make it your own!

Strawberry Banana Protein Sorbet

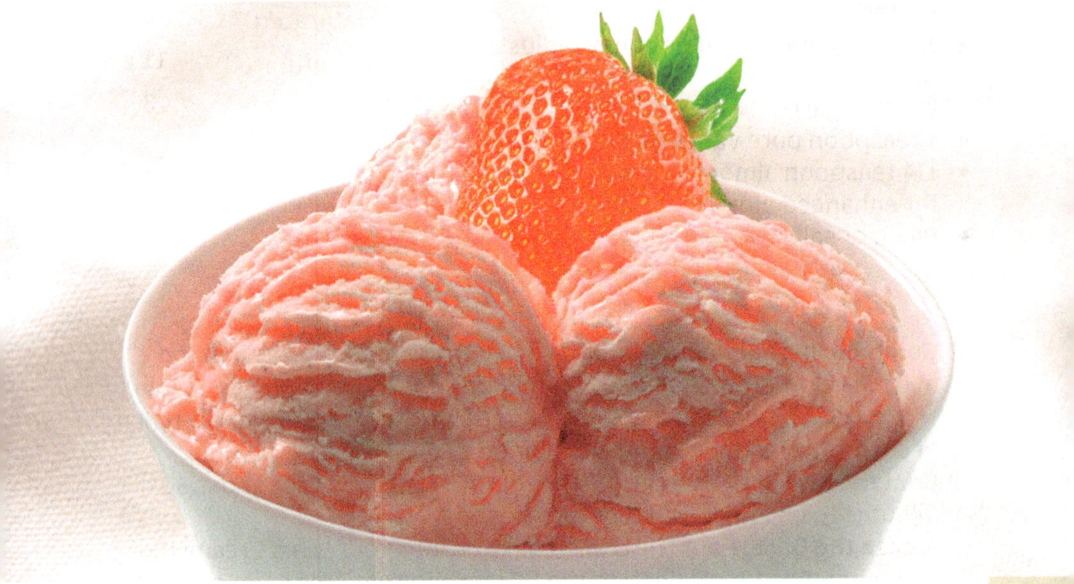

The Strawberry Banana Protein Sorbet is a refreshing and fruity treat that combines two classic flavors into a delightful frozen dessert. This recipe is not only incredibly simple to make but also packed with nutrients, making it a perfect post-workout snack or a healthy dessert option for the whole family. The natural sweetness of ripe strawberries and bananas provides a delicious base, while the addition of protein powder ensures you're getting a good boost of protein to help with muscle recovery. I often prepare this sorbet for my daughter, Emma, who loves the vibrant colors and fruity flavors. It's a great way to enjoy a guilt-free indulgence!

Ingredients

- 2 cups fresh strawberries, hulled and sliced (or frozen strawberries, thawed)
- 1 ripe banana, sliced (fresh or frozen)
- 1 cup unsweetened almond milk (or any milk of choice)
- 1 scoop vanilla protein powder (whey or plant-based)
- 1 tablespoon honey or maple syrup (optional, adjust to taste)
- Juice of 1 lemon (about 2 tablespoons)
- Pinch of salt

Nutrition

Calories	150
Protein	10 g
Carbohydrates	35 g
Sugars	20 g
Fats (Total)	1 g
Saturated	0 g
Unsaturated	1 g
Fiber	3 g

Instructions

1. **Prepare the Fruit:** If using fresh strawberries, rinse them under cold water and hull them. If using frozen strawberries, allow them to thaw slightly for easier blending.
2. **Blend the Mixture:** In a blender, combine the strawberries, banana, almond milk, protein powder, honey (if using), lemon juice, and a pinch of salt. Blend until smooth and creamy.
3. **Taste and Adjust:** Taste the mixture and adjust sweetness if necessary by adding more honey or maple syrup. Blend again if you make any adjustments.
4. **Freeze the Mixture:** Pour the blended mixture into your Ninja Creami pint container. Ensure it's filled to the fill line and then freeze for at least 24 hours.

Creami Processing

1. **Creami Processing:** After freezing, remove the pint from the freezer. Place it in your Ninja Creami machine, select the "Sorbet" function, and process until smooth.
2. **Serve or Store:** Enjoy immediately for a refreshing soft-serve texture or return to the freezer for a firmer consistency. You can also garnish with extra sliced strawberries or a sprinkle of granola for added crunch.

Nutritionist Tips

- **Flavor Variations:** Feel free to experiment with other fruits such as mango or peach for a tropical twist. You can also add a handful of spinach for an extra nutrient boost without affecting the flavor significantly.

Mint Chocolate Chip Protein Ice Cream

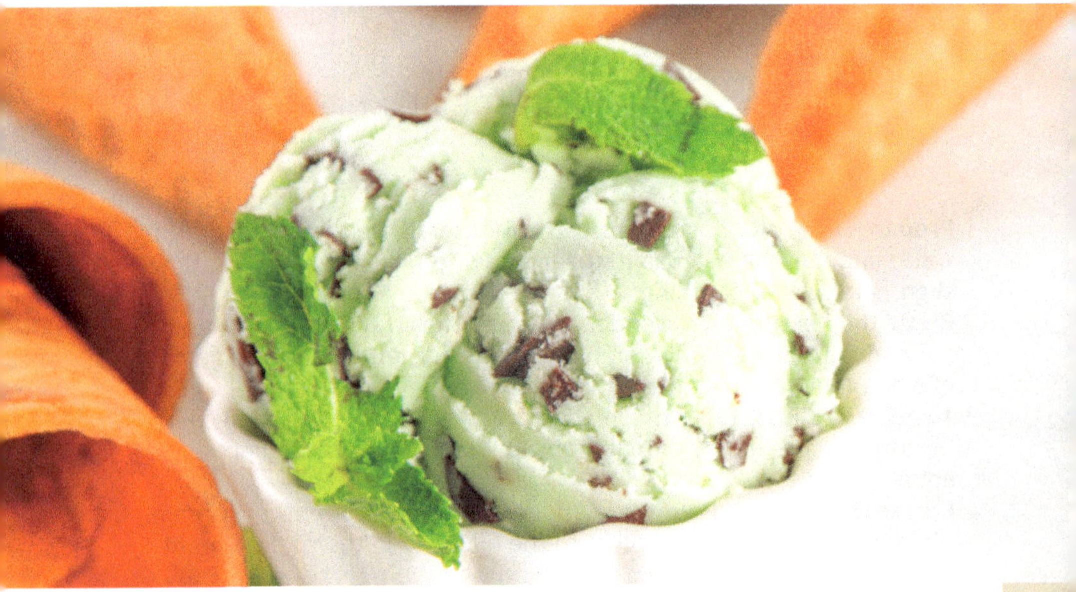

The Mint Chocolate Chip Protein Ice Cream is a refreshing and indulgent treat that beautifully marries the coolness of mint with the rich flavor of chocolate. This recipe is perfect for those warm days when you crave something sweet yet healthful. The addition of protein powder makes it an excellent choice for a post-workout recovery or a nutritious dessert that satisfies your cravings. I love making this ice cream for my family, especially during the summer months, as it's a fantastic way to enjoy a classic flavor while boosting our protein intake. With its vibrant green color and delightful chocolate chips, this ice cream is sure to be a hit!

Ingredients

- 2 cups unsweetened almond milk (or any milk of choice)
- 1 cup plain Greek yogurt (non-fat or full-fat based on preference)
- 1/2 cup vanilla protein powder (whey or plant-based)
- 1/4 cup granulated sugar or your preferred sweetener (adjust to taste; can use agave syrup or erythritol for lower sugar)
- 1 teaspoon pure peppermint extract (adjust based on preference)
- A few drops of green food coloring (optional, for a vibrant color)
- 1/4 cup mini dark chocolate chips (dairy-free if needed)
- Pinch of salt

Nutrition

Calories	**210**
Protein	**20 g**
Carbohydrates	**15 g**
Sugars	**5 g**
Fats (Total)	**6 g**
Saturated	**2 g**
Unsaturated	**4 g**
Fiber	**1 g**

Instructions

1. **Combine Ingredients:** In a mixing bowl, whisk together the almond milk, Greek yogurt, protein powder, granulated sugar (or sweetener), peppermint extract, and a pinch of salt until smooth and well combined. If using, add a few drops of green food coloring to achieve your desired shade of mint green.
2. **Cool the Mixture:** Chill the mixture in the refrigerator for about 30 minutes to ensure it's cold before freezing.
3. **Freeze the Base:** Pour the chilled mixture into your Ninja Creami pint container. Ensure it's filled to the fill line and then freeze for at least 24 hours.

Creami Processing

1. **Creami Processing:** After freezing, remove the pint from the freezer. Place it in your Ninja Creami machine, select the "Ice Cream" function, and process until smooth and creamy.
2. **Add Chocolate Chips:** Gently fold in the mini chocolate chips after processing for an even distribution throughout the ice cream.
3. **Serve or Store:** Enjoy immediately for a soft-serve texture or return to the freezer for a firmer consistency. For an extra special touch, garnish with additional chocolate chips or a sprig of fresh mint before serving.

Healthy
SNACKS & TREATS

Protein-Packed Popsicles

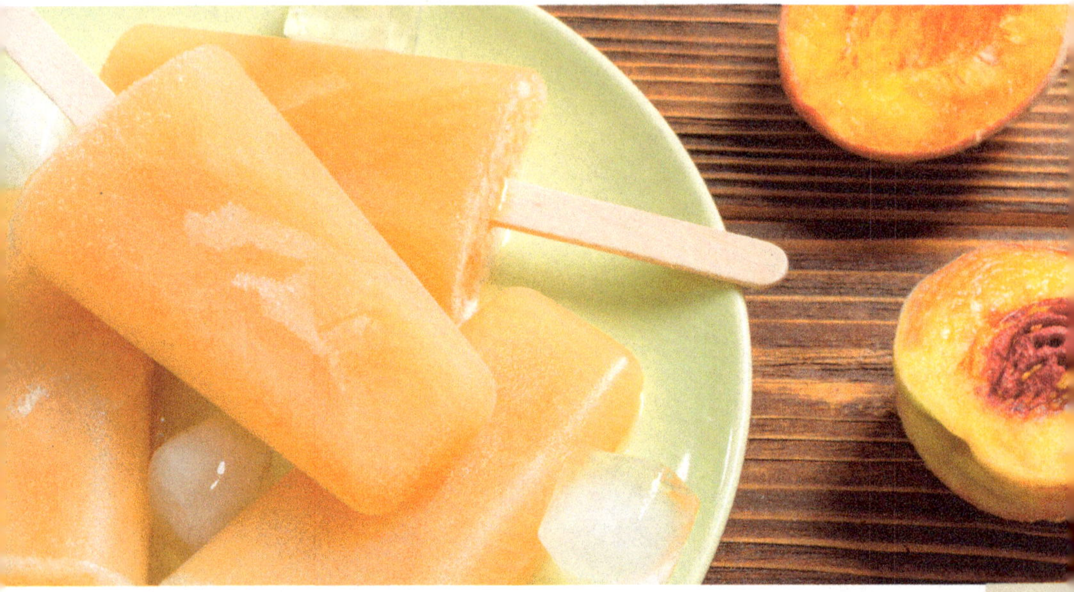

These Protein-Packed Popsicles are a fantastic way to enjoy a refreshing treat while boosting your protein intake. Perfect for hot summer days or after a workout, these popsicles are made with wholesome ingredients that keep you feeling satisfied and nourished. The combination of fruits, yogurt, and protein powder creates a deliciously creamy texture that's both healthy and indulgent. I love making these popsicles with my daughter, Emma, as they're easy to prepare and a fun way to experiment with different flavor combinations. They're not only a hit with kids but also a great way to sneak in extra nutrients!

Ingredients

- 1 cup unsweetened almond milk (or any milk of choice)
- 1 cup plain Greek yogurt (non-fat or full-fat based on preference)
- 1/2 cup fruit puree (such as strawberries, mangoes, or peaches)
- 1 scoop vanilla or fruit-flavored protein powder (whey or plant-based)
- 2 tablespoons honey or maple syrup (optional, adjust to taste)
- Fresh fruit pieces (optional, for added texture)

Nutrition

Calories	**90**
Protein	**6 g**
Carbohydrates	**12 g**
Sugars	**5 g**
Fats (Total)	**3 g**
Saturated	**1.5 g**
Unsaturated	**1.5 g**
Fiber	**0 g**

Instructions

1. **Combine Ingredients:** In a mixing bowl, whisk together the almond milk, Greek yogurt, fruit puree, protein powder, and honey (if using) until smooth and well combined.
2. **Taste and Adjust:** Taste the mixture and adjust sweetness if necessary by adding more honey or maple syrup. Blend again if you make any adjustments.
3. **Prepare the Popsicle Molds:** If you want to add fresh fruit pieces, place a few pieces at the bottom of each popsicle mold.
4. **Fill the Molds:** Pour the mixture evenly into the popsicle molds, leaving a little space at the top as the mixture will expand while freezing.
5. **Insert Sticks:** If your molds have lids, insert the sticks according to the manufacturer's instructions. If not, wait for about 30 minutes until the popsicles start to freeze slightly, then insert the sticks.
6. **Freeze:** Place the molds in the freezer and freeze for at least 4-6 hours or until completely solid.
7. **Unmold and Serve:** To remove the popsicles, run warm water over the outside of the molds for a few seconds. Gently pull on the sticks to release the popsicles. Enjoy immediately!

Nutritionist Tips

- **Fruit Puree:** Use fresh or frozen fruits to make your own puree. Simply blend the fruit until smooth and strain if desired for a smoother texture.

Protein Energy Bites

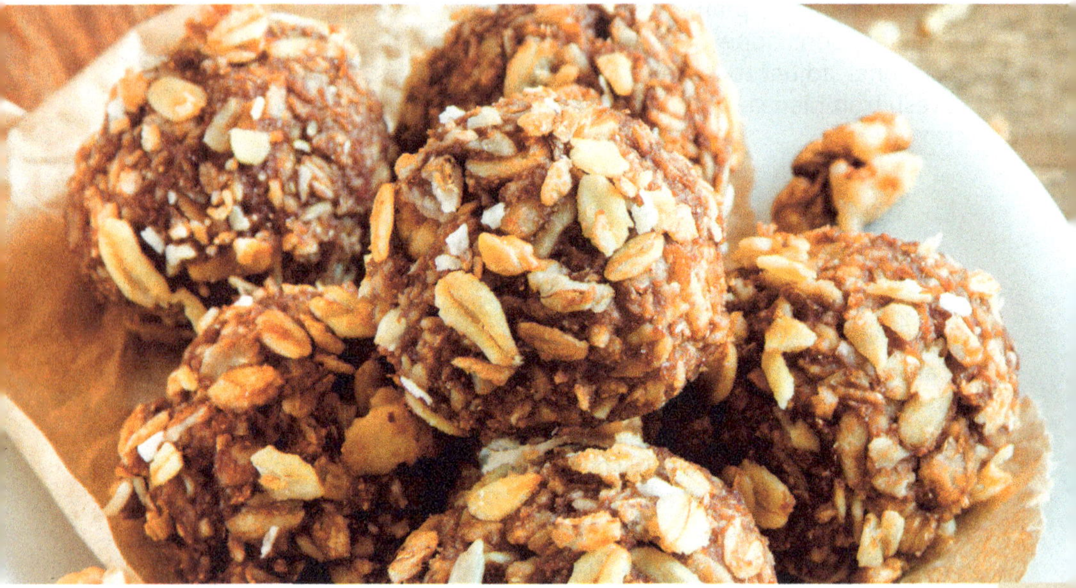

These Protein Energy Bites are a fantastic on-the-go snack that combines convenience with nutrition. Packed with protein and healthy fats, they are perfect for a quick pick-me-up before a workout or as a satisfying treat any time of the day. I created this recipe to help my family enjoy a nutritious snack that's also delicious and easy to prepare. With a delightful blend of oats, nut butter, and chocolate chips, these bites are not only energizing but also satisfy that craving for something sweet. They're a hit with my daughter, Emma, who loves to help roll them into bite-sized pieces!

Ingredients

- 1 cup rolled oats (use gluten-free oats if needed)
- 1/2 cup natural nut butter (such as almond butter or peanut butter)
- 1/2 cup honey or maple syrup (or a low-carb sweetener for a sugar-free option)
- 1/2 cup protein powder (vanilla or chocolate)
- 1/4 cup mini chocolate chips (dairy-free if needed)
- 1/4 cup chopped nuts or seeds (optional, for added crunch)
- 1 teaspoon vanilla extract
- Pinch of salt

Nutrition

Calories	**120**
Protein	**5 g**
Carbohydrates	**15 g**
Sugars	**5 g**
Fats (Total)	**5 g**
Saturated	**1 g**
Unsaturated	**4 g**
Fiber	**2 g**

Instructions

1. **Combine Ingredients:** In a large mixing bowl, combine the rolled oats, nut butter, honey (or sweetener), protein powder, mini chocolate chips, chopped nuts or seeds (if using), vanilla extract, and a pinch of salt.
2. **Mix Well:** Using a spatula or your hands, mix all the ingredients together until fully combined. The mixture should be sticky and hold together well. If it's too dry, add a little more nut butter or honey; if it's too wet, add a bit more oats or protein powder.
3. **Chill the Mixture:** Cover the bowl and refrigerate the mixture for about 30 minutes. Chilling makes it easier to roll into bites.
4. **Form the Bites:** Once chilled, take about a tablespoon of the mixture and roll it into a ball. Place the balls on a parchment-lined baking sheet or plate. Repeat until all the mixture is used.
5. **Store:** You can enjoy the protein energy bites immediately, or store them in an airtight container in the refrigerator for up to one week. They can also be frozen for longer storage—just thaw them before enjoying!

Nutritionist Tips

- **Texture Variations:** Feel free to add in other mix-ins like dried fruits, coconut flakes, or seeds for added texture and flavor.
- **Portion Control:** These bites are easy to grab and go, but be mindful of portion sizes, especially if you're watching your caloric intake.

Coconut Protein Bark

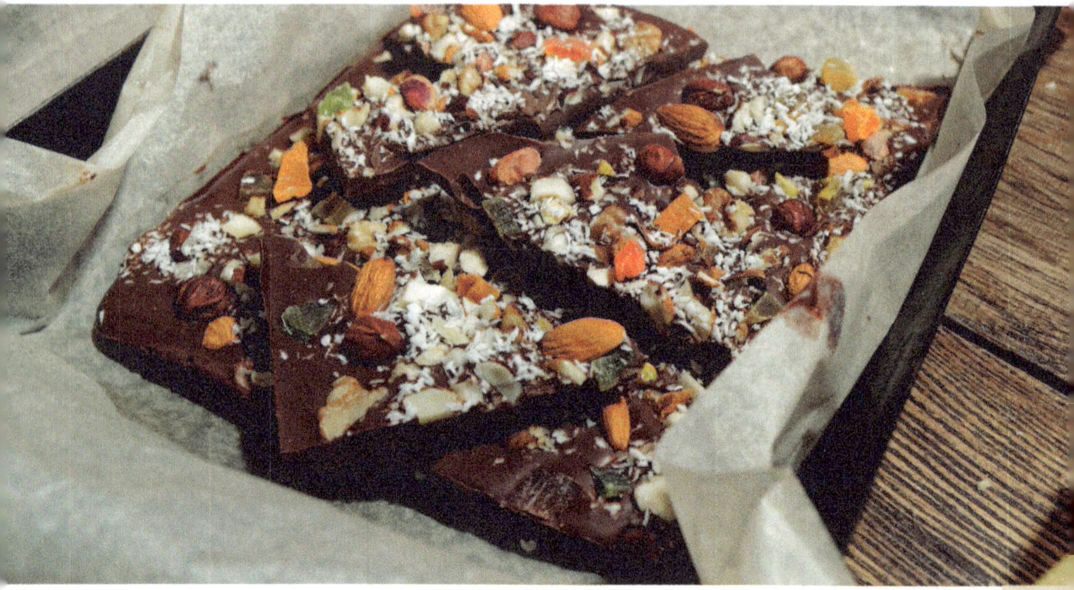

The Coconut Protein Bark is a delightful and nutritious treat that combines the tropical flavor of coconut with the satisfying crunch of dark chocolate. This recipe is perfect for satisfying your sweet cravings while providing a healthy dose of protein and healthy fats. I created this bark as a quick snack option that my family can enjoy at any time of the day, whether it's a post-workout boost or a sweet treat after dinner. It's incredibly easy to make, and you can customize it with your favorite toppings to create a truly unique flavor experience!

Ingredients

- 1 cup dark chocolate chips (dairy-free if preferred)
- 1/4 cup coconut oil
- 1/2 cup vanilla or chocolate protein powder (whey or plant-based)
- 1 cup unsweetened shredded coconut
- 1/4 cup chopped nuts (such as almonds or walnuts, optional)
- 1/4 cup dried fruit (such as cranberries or apricots, optional)
- Pinch of sea salt

Nutrition

Calories	150
Protein	5 g
Carbohydrates	12 g
Sugars	6 g
Fats (Total)	10 g
Saturated	6 g
Unsaturated	4 g
Fiber	2 g

Instructions

1. **Melt Chocolate and Coconut Oil:** In a microwave-safe bowl, combine the dark chocolate chips and coconut oil. Microwave in 30-second intervals, stirring in between, until completely melted and smooth.
2. **Mix in Protein Powder:** Once melted, remove the bowl from the microwave and stir in the protein powder until fully combined. The mixture will thicken as you mix.
3. **Add Coconut and Nuts:** Gently fold in the shredded coconut, chopped nuts, and dried fruit (if using) until evenly distributed throughout the chocolate mixture.
4. **Prepare the Baking Sheet:** Line a baking sheet or a shallow dish with parchment paper. Pour the chocolate mixture onto the prepared sheet and spread it out evenly with a spatula to your desired thickness.
5. **Sprinkle with Sea Salt:** Lightly sprinkle a pinch of sea salt on top for added flavor.
6. **Refrigerate:** Place the baking sheet in the refrigerator for about 1-2 hours, or until the chocolate is fully set and hardened.
7. **Break Into Pieces:** Once set, remove the bark from the refrigerator and break it into pieces of your desired size.
8. **Store:** Store the coconut protein bark in an airtight container in the refrigerator for up to two weeks.

Nutritionist Tips

- **Coconut Variations:** For extra coconut flavor, use toasted shredded coconut or add a few drops of coconut extract to the mixture.

Frozen Yogurt Bark with Berries

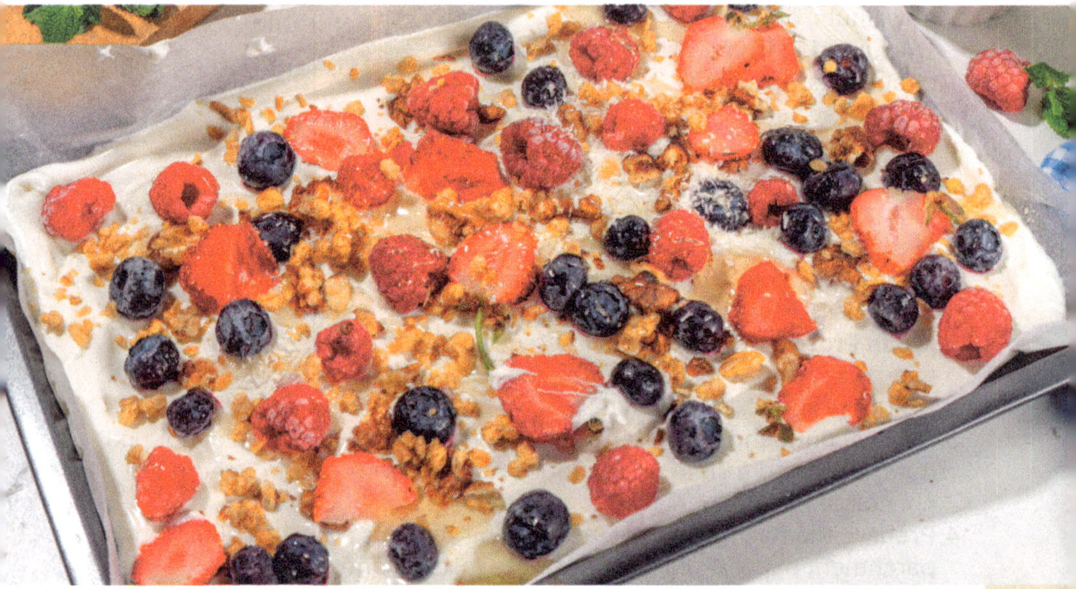

The Frozen Yogurt Bark with Berries is a delightful and healthful treat that's perfect for warm days or as a quick, nutritious snack. This recipe combines creamy yogurt with the vibrant flavors of fresh berries, creating a visually appealing and delicious dessert that the whole family will love. I often prepare this bark as a fun way to get my daughter, Emma, involved in the kitchen. It's simple to make, customizable with your favorite toppings, and a fantastic way to enjoy the natural sweetness of fruit while reaping the benefits of probiotics from yogurt. This frozen dessert is not only refreshing but also a great way to satisfy your sweet tooth without guilt!

Ingredients

- 2 cups plain Greek yogurt (non-fat or full-fat based on preference)
- 2 tablespoons honey or maple syrup (adjust to taste; can use sugar-free sweetener for lower sugar)
- 1 teaspoon pure vanilla extract
- 1 cup mixed fresh berries (such as strawberries, blueberries, raspberries, and blackberries)
- Optional toppings: shredded coconut, chopped nuts, or granola

Nutrition

Calories	**80**
Protein	**5 g**
Carbohydrates	**11 g**
Sugars	**6 g**
Fats (Total)	**2 g**
Saturated	**1 g**
Unsaturated	**1 g**
Fiber	**1 g**

Instructions

1. **Prepare the Yogurt Mixture:** In a mixing bowl, combine the Greek yogurt, honey (or sweetener), and vanilla extract. Stir until well mixed and smooth.
2. **Line the Baking Sheet:** Line a baking sheet or a shallow dish with parchment paper, ensuring it covers the bottom completely for easy removal later.
3. **Spread the Yogurt:** Pour the yogurt mixture onto the prepared baking sheet. Use a spatula to spread it evenly to your desired thickness, typically about 1/4 inch thick.
4. **Add Berries:** Evenly distribute the mixed fresh berries over the yogurt layer, pressing them down slightly to ensure they stick. If desired, sprinkle with any optional toppings like shredded coconut or chopped nuts for added texture.
5. **Freeze:** Place the baking sheet in the freezer and freeze for at least 4 hours or until the yogurt is completely firm.
6. **Break into Pieces:** Once fully frozen, remove the bark from the freezer. Lift the parchment paper to remove the yogurt bark from the baking sheet and break it into pieces of your desired size.
7. **Store:** Store the frozen yogurt bark pieces in an airtight container in the freezer for up to two weeks.

Nutritionist Tips

- **Yogurt Choice:** Opt for plain Greek yogurt for a protein boost and a tangy flavor. If you prefer a sweeter taste, consider using flavored yogurt, but be mindful of added sugars.
- **Berry Selection:** Use a mix of your favorite berries for a colorful, nutritious treat. If fresh berries are not available, frozen berries can work as well—just ensure they're thawed and drained before use.

Creative PROTEIN DESSERTS

Protein-Packed Chia Seed Pudding

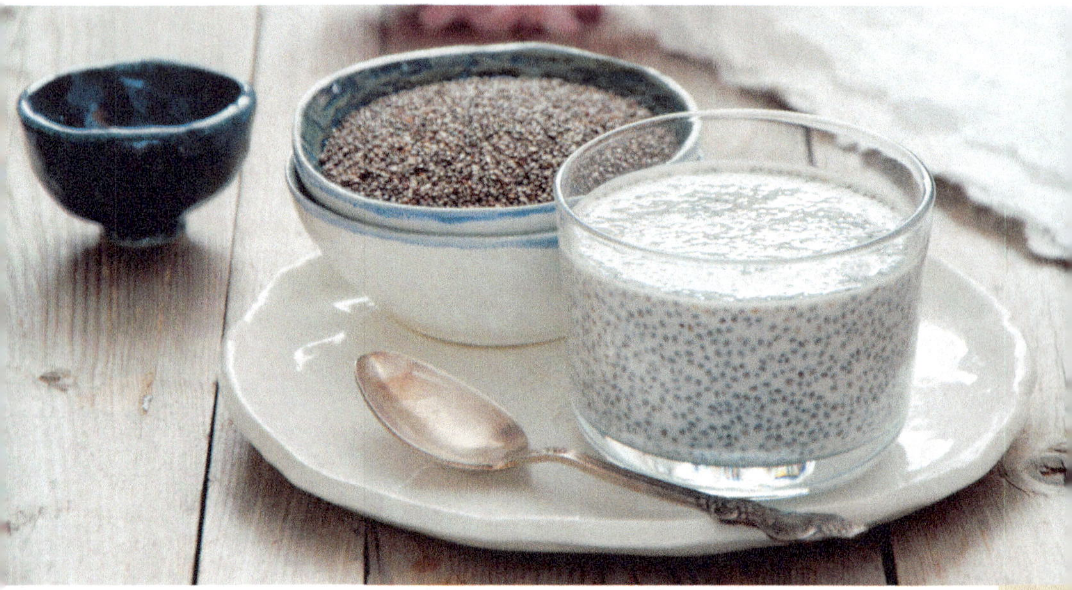

The Protein-Packed Chia Seed Pudding is a versatile and nutritious treat that I absolutely love for breakfast or as a snack! Chia seeds are tiny nutritional powerhouses, rich in omega-3 fatty acids, fiber, and protein, making them an ideal ingredient for a health-conscious diet. This pudding is creamy, satisfying, and incredibly easy to prepare. With just a few simple ingredients, you can create a delightful dessert that can be customized with your favorite flavors and toppings. I often prepare this pudding in advance, allowing my family to enjoy a quick and nutritious option that is both delicious and filling. It's a fantastic way to incorporate more healthy fats and protein into your diet while satisfying your sweet tooth!

Ingredients

- 1/2 cup chia seeds
- 2 cups unsweetened almond milk (or any milk of choice)
- 1/4 cup vanilla protein powder (whey or plant-based)
- 2 tablespoons maple syrup or honey (adjust to taste; can use sugar-free sweetener for lower sugar)
- 1 teaspoon vanilla extract
- A pinch of salt
- Optional toppings: fresh fruits, nuts, granola, or shredded coconut

Nutrition

Calories	180
Protein	10 g
Carbohydrates	24 g
Sugars	6 g
Fats (Total)	7 g
Saturated	0.5 g
Unsaturated	6.5 g
Fiber	10 g

Instructions

1. **Combine Ingredients:** In a mixing bowl, whisk together the almond milk, vanilla protein powder, maple syrup (or honey), vanilla extract, chia seeds, and a pinch of salt until well combined.
2. **Let It Sit:** Allow the mixture to sit for about 5 minutes, then whisk again to prevent the chia seeds from clumping together.
3. **Refrigerate:** Cover the bowl with plastic wrap or transfer the mixture to individual serving jars. Refrigerate for at least 4 hours or overnight. The chia seeds will absorb the liquid and thicken into a pudding-like consistency.
4. **Serve:** Once the pudding has thickened, give it a good stir before serving. If it's too thick, you can add a splash of milk to reach your desired consistency.
5. **Add Toppings:** Top with your choice of fresh fruits, nuts, granola, or shredded coconut for added flavor and texture.

Nutritionist Tips

- **Chia Seed Benefits:** Chia seeds are not only high in protein but also packed with fiber, which aids in digestion and helps you feel full longer. They also absorb liquid, creating a gel-like texture that is perfect for puddings.
- **Milk Alternatives:** Feel free to use any milk that fits your dietary preferences—coconut milk will add a rich flavor, while oat milk can provide a creamier consistency.
- **Flavor Variations:** Experiment with different flavors by adding cocoa powder for a chocolate version, or blend in pureed fruits like mango or banana for a fruity twist.

Nutty Protein Granola

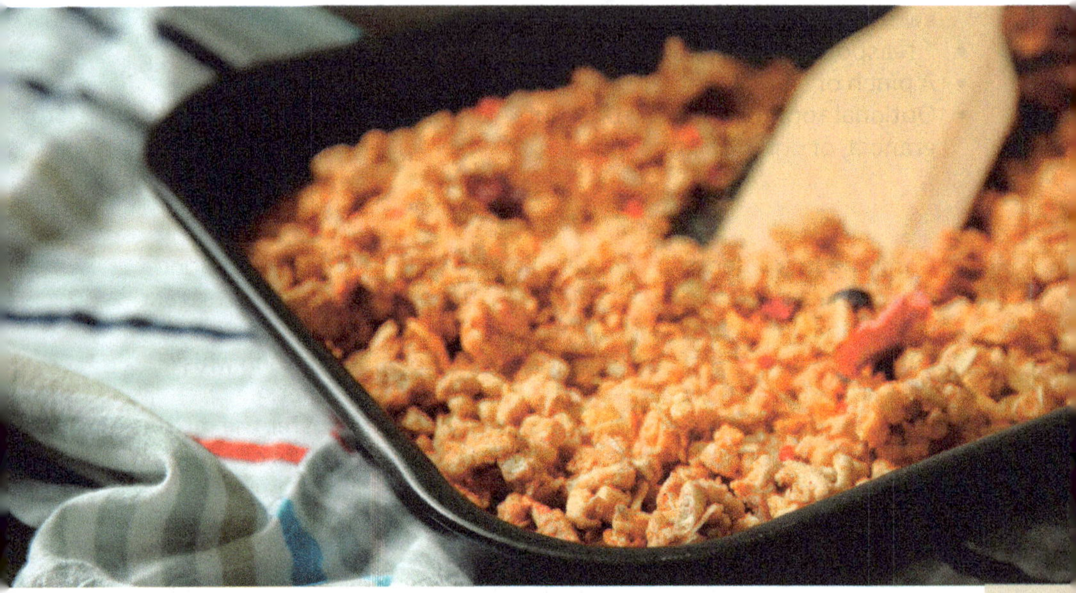

The Nutty Protein Granola is a wholesome and satisfying snack that's perfect for breakfast or as a crunchy topping for yogurt and smoothies. Packed with a variety of nuts, seeds, and protein powder, this granola not only provides a delightful crunch but also fuels your day with essential nutrients. I created this recipe to help my family enjoy a nutritious option that is both delicious and easy to prepare. It's a versatile treat that can be customized with your favorite flavors and ingredients. I love making a big batch to keep on hand for busy mornings or when we need a quick energy boost during the day!

Ingredients

- 2 cups rolled oats (use gluten-free oats if needed)
- 1/2 cup chopped nuts (such as almonds, walnuts, or pecans)
- 1/2 cup mixed seeds (such as pumpkin seeds, sunflower seeds, or chia seeds)
- 1/2 cup nut butter (such as almond butter or peanut butter)
- 1/4 cup honey or maple syrup (adjust to taste; can use sugar-free sweetener for lower sugar)
- 1/4 cup vanilla protein powder (whey or plant-based)
- 1 teaspoon cinnamon
- 1/2 teaspoon vanilla extract
- Pinch of salt

Nutrition

Calories	**200**
Protein	**8 g**
Carbohydrates	**24 g**
Sugars	**7 g**
Fats (Total)	**10 g**
Saturated	**2 g**
Unsaturated	**8 g**
Fiber	**3 g**

Instructions

1. **Preheat the Oven:** Preheat your oven to 350°F (175°C) and line a baking sheet with parchment paper.
2. **Combine Dry Ingredients:** In a large mixing bowl, combine the rolled oats, chopped nuts, mixed seeds, protein powder, cinnamon, and a pinch of salt. Mix well to ensure even distribution of the dry ingredients.
3. **Mix Wet Ingredients:** In a separate bowl, combine the nut butter and honey (or maple syrup). If the nut butter is too thick, you may need to warm it slightly in the microwave for easier mixing. Stir in the vanilla extract until smooth.
4. **Combine Mixtures:** Pour the wet mixture over the dry ingredients and stir until everything is well coated and combined.
5. **Spread on Baking Sheet:** Transfer the granola mixture to the prepared baking sheet and spread it out evenly.
6. **Bake:** Bake in the preheated oven for about 20-25 minutes, stirring halfway through to ensure even browning. Keep an eye on it to prevent burning; the granola should be golden brown when done.
7. **Cool:** Remove from the oven and let the granola cool completely on the baking sheet. It will become crisp as it cools.
8. **Store:** Once cooled, break the granola into clusters and transfer it to an airtight container. Store at room temperature for up to two weeks.

Layered Yogurt Parfait

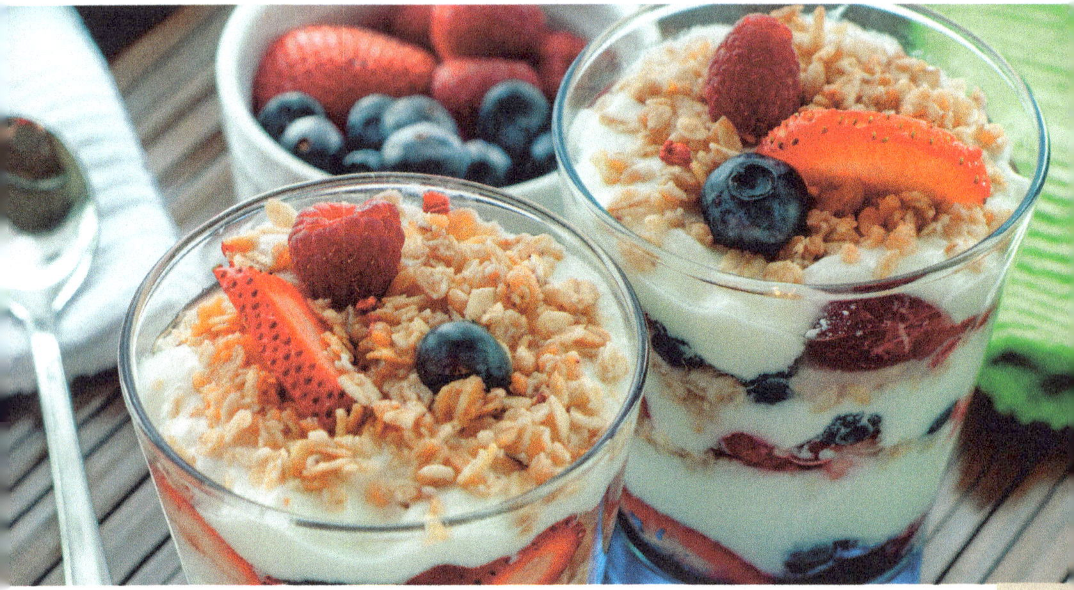

The Layered Yogurt Parfait is a delightful and visually appealing treat that combines creamy yogurt with layers of fresh fruits and crunchy granola. It's a perfect option for breakfast, a snack, or even a light dessert. This recipe is incredibly versatile, allowing you to use whatever fruits and toppings you have on hand, making it easy to customize for different seasons or dietary preferences. I love preparing this parfait for my family, especially Emma, who enjoys helping to layer the ingredients. It's not only delicious but also packed with protein, fiber, and essential nutrients, making it a guilt-free indulgence that everyone can enjoy!

Ingredients

- 2 cups plain Greek yogurt (non-fat or full-fat based on preference)
- 1 cup mixed fresh berries (such as strawberries, blueberries, raspberries, and blackberries)
- 1/2 cup granola (store-bought or homemade)
- 2 tablespoons honey or maple syrup (optional, adjust to taste)
- 1 teaspoon vanilla extract (optional)
- Additional toppings: sliced almonds, chia seeds, or shredded coconut (optional)

Nutrition

Calories	**180**
Protein	**12 g**
Carbohydrates	**25 g**
Sugars	**10 g**
Fats (Total)	**5 g**
Saturated	**2 g**
Unsaturated	**3 g**
Fiber	**3 g**

Instructions

1. **Prepare the Yogurt:** In a mixing bowl, combine the Greek yogurt, honey (if using), and vanilla extract (if using). Stir well until smooth and creamy.
2. **Prepare the Fruit:** Wash and slice the fresh berries as needed. If using larger fruits like strawberries, slice them into smaller pieces for layering.
3. **Layer the Parfait:** In serving glasses or bowls, start by adding a layer of the yogurt mixture at the bottom. Follow with a layer of mixed berries, then add a layer of granola. Repeat the layers until the glasses are filled, finishing with a layer of yogurt on top.
4. **Top and Garnish:** If desired, garnish the top with additional berries, a sprinkle of granola, and any other toppings such as sliced almonds or shredded coconut.
5. **Serve:** Enjoy immediately, or refrigerate for up to 2 hours if you prefer a chilled parfait. If storing, keep the granola separate until ready to serve to maintain its crunch.

Nutritionist Tips

- **Yogurt Selection:** Greek yogurt is a great source of protein and adds creaminess to the parfait. You can also use plant-based yogurt if you prefer a dairy-free option.
- **Granola Choices:** Choose a granola that is low in added sugars and high in whole grains. You can also make your own granola for a healthier option.

Hi There!

I hope you are enjoying my book so far. I would really appreciate it if you could leave a quick review on Amazon.

Just simply scan the code below using your mobile phone's camera, or you can enter the link below on our web browser.

https://swiy.com/ReviewCreami3

Thanks a lot!

- Clara

MEAL PREP AND PLANNING

Quick Meal Prep Tips
for Busy Lifestyles

In today's fast-paced world, effective meal prep can be a game changer for maintaining a healthy diet, especially when it comes to incorporating protein-rich recipes into your daily routine. Here are some practical tips to help you streamline your meal prep and ensure you always have nutritious options on hand:

Schedule Your Prep Time
Set aside a specific day each week for meal prep. This could be on the weekends or a day that works best for you. Planning ahead will help you stay organized and make healthier choices throughout the week.

Batch Cooking
Prepare larger quantities of staple items such as grains, proteins, and vegetables in one go. This allows you to mix and match components throughout the week, saving time and ensuring variety in your meals.

Utilize Freezer-Friendly Recipes
Make use of your freezer by preparing protein-rich frozen treats, soups, and smoothies in advance. Portion them into containers or bags for easy access during busy days. The Ninja Creami is perfect for this, allowing you to whip up delicious frozen snacks quickly.

Keep It Simple
Focus on simple recipes that require minimal ingredients and preparation time. The easier the recipe, the more likely you are to stick with your meal prep routine.

Label and Organize

Label containers with the contents and date of preparation. This will help you keep track of what you have on hand and ensure you consume items before they spoil.

Involve the Family

Make meal prep a family affair! Get your kids involved by having them help wash and chop vegetables or assemble snacks. This not only teaches them valuable cooking skills but also makes healthy eating a fun activity.

Plan for Snacks

Don't forget to include snacks in your meal prep! Prepare protein-packed energy bites, yogurt parfaits, or fruit and nut mixes to have on hand for quick, nutritious options.

How to Create Your Own Protein-Rich Meal Plans

Creating a protein-rich meal plan can help you meet your nutritional goals while ensuring you enjoy a variety of flavors and textures. Here's how to get started:

1. **Assess Your Protein Needs:** Determine how much protein you need based on your age, activity level, and health goals. A general guideline is to aim for about 0.8 grams of protein per kilogram of body weight, while athletes may require more.

2. **Choose a Variety of Protein Sources:** Include a mix of animal and plant-based proteins in your meal plan. Options include lean meats, poultry, fish, eggs, dairy, legumes, nuts, seeds, and protein powders. This variety helps ensure you get a balanced intake of essential amino acids.

3. **Plan Balanced Meals:** Each meal should include a source of protein, healthy fats, and carbohydrates. For example, pair grilled chicken with quinoa and a side of roasted vegetables, or enjoy a smoothie made with Greek yogurt, fruit, and protein powder.

4. **Create a Weekly Menu:** Write down your meals for the week, including breakfast, lunch, dinner, and snacks. This will help you stay organized and ensure you're incorporating enough protein each day.

5. **Grocery List:** Based on your meal plan, create a grocery list that includes all the ingredients you'll need. This will make shopping more efficient and help you avoid impulse buys.

6. **Prep Ahead:** Cook and prepare protein-rich ingredients in advance. For instance, grill a batch of chicken breasts, cook quinoa, or roast chickpeas at the beginning of the week to have ready for quick meal assembly.

7. **Stay Flexible:** Life can be unpredictable, so be prepared to adjust your meal plan as needed. If you have leftovers, incorporate them into your next day's meals to minimize waste and save time.

By implementing these meal prep tips and strategies for creating a protein-rich meal plan, you can simplify your cooking process and ensure that you and your family enjoy nutritious meals throughout the week. Let's dive into the exciting recipes that will help you maximize your health while indulging in delicious frozen treats!

SHOPPING MADE SIMPLE

Essential Ingredients to Stock for Protein Recipes

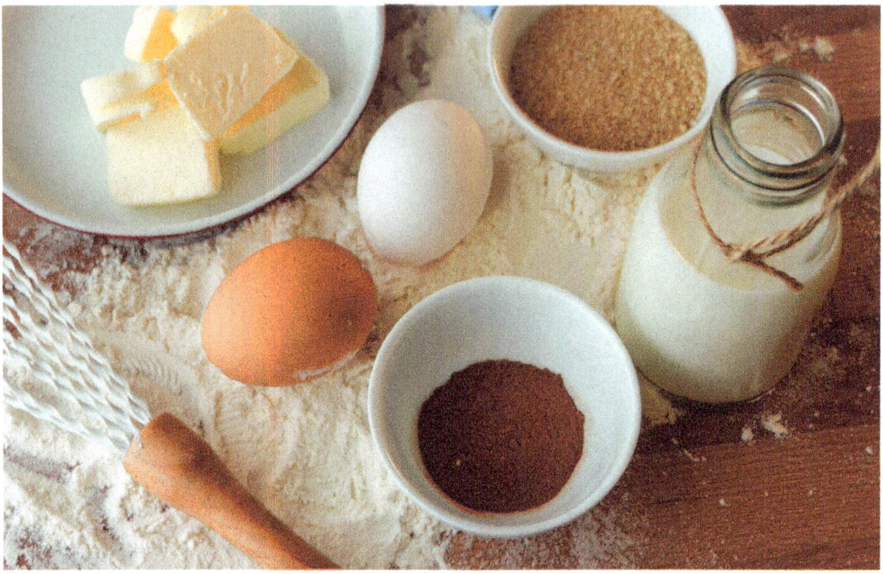

To make your meal preparation seamless and efficient, it's essential to have a well-stocked pantry and refrigerator with key ingredients that support high-protein recipes. Here's a list of must-have items to ensure you can whip up nutritious and delicious meals and snacks anytime:

Protein Powders

- Whey Protein: A complete protein source that is easily digestible and perfect for shakes, smoothies, and baked goods.
- Plant-Based Protein: Options like pea, hemp, or brown rice protein are excellent for those who prefer a vegan or dairy-free option.

Greek Yogurt

- A versatile ingredient that provides a creamy texture and high protein content. It can be used in smoothies, parfaits, or as a base for frozen treats.

Nut Butters

- Almond butter, peanut butter, or sunflower seed butter provide healthy fats and protein. These can be added to smoothies, energy bites, or used as a spread.

Cottage Cheese

- A great source of protein that can be enjoyed on its own, mixed into smoothies, or used in various recipes for added creaminess.

Legumes

- Canned or dried beans, lentils, and chickpeas are excellent plant-based protein sources that can be added to salads, soups, and snacks.

Nuts and Seeds

- Almonds, walnuts, chia seeds, and pumpkin seeds offer healthy fats, protein, and fiber. They can be used in granola, smoothies, or as toppings for yogurt and desserts.

Dairy Alternatives

- Unsweetened almond milk, coconut milk, and oat milk can be used as bases for smoothies, shakes, and frozen desserts.

Whole Grains

- Quinoa, brown rice, and rolled oats are great sources of protein and can serve as the foundation for many meals and snacks.

Fresh and Frozen Fruits

- Berries, bananas, mangoes, and other fruits provide natural sweetness and essential vitamins. They are perfect for smoothies, toppings, and desserts.

Healthy Oils

- Coconut oil and olive oil can be used in cooking and baking, adding flavor and healthy fats to your meals.

Where to Find
Healthy Protein Ingredients

Finding high-quality protein ingredients is key to preparing nutritious meals and snacks. Here are some tips on where to shop for these essential items:

1. **Local Grocery Stores:** Most grocery stores carry a variety of protein-rich foods, including fresh meats, dairy, and plant-based options. Look for organic or grass-fed options when possible for added nutritional benefits.
2. **Health Food Stores:** These stores typically have a wider selection of specialty items, such as protein powders, non-dairy yogurts, and organic grains. They are excellent resources for finding high-quality ingredients that support your health goals.
3. **Farmers' Markets:** Fresh produce, eggs, and local meats can often be found at farmers' markets, providing you with high-quality ingredients while supporting local agriculture. This is also a great way to find seasonal fruits and vegetables.
4. **Online Retailers:** Consider purchasing bulk items like nuts, seeds, and protein powders from reputable online retailers. This can also be a convenient option for specialty items that may not be available locally.
5. **Specialty Health Websites:** Websites dedicated to health and wellness often offer a variety of high-quality protein-rich products, from superfoods to supplements. Look for trusted brands with positive reviews.
6. **Warehouse Clubs:** Stores like Costco or Sam's Club can provide bulk options for many healthy ingredients at a lower price point, making it easy to stock up on essentials.

By stocking your kitchen with these essential ingredients and knowing where to find them, you'll be well-prepared to create delicious and protein-rich recipes using your Ninja Creami.

TIPS FOR SUCCESS

Navigating Social Situations with Healthy Treats

Maintaining healthy eating habits can be particularly challenging in social situations, where indulgent foods often take center stage. However, with some planning and strategies, you can enjoy gatherings while staying true to your health goals. Here are some tips to help you navigate social situations with confidence:

- **Bring Your Own Treats:** If you're attending a party or gathering, consider bringing a healthy dessert or snack that you can enjoy. This not only ensures you have something nutritious to indulge in but also introduces others to delicious healthy options. Recipes from the **Ninja Creami Protein Cookbook** are perfect for this!

- **Make Smart Choices:** When faced with a buffet or dessert table, take a moment to assess your options. Look for healthier choices like fruit salads, yogurt parfaits, or dark chocolate. If you choose to indulge, opt for smaller portions to keep your overall intake balanced.

- **Communicate Your Goals:** Don't hesitate to share your dietary preferences or goals with friends and family. Many people are supportive and will appreciate your commitment to healthy eating. You may even inspire them to join you in making healthier choices!

- **Stay Mindful:** Practice mindful eating by savoring each bite and enjoying the flavors of the food. This can help you feel satisfied with smaller portions and reduce the likelihood of overindulging.

Involving Family in the Kitchen:

Fun Activities for Kids

Cooking together is a wonderful way to bond as a family and teach children valuable skills about healthy eating. Here are some fun activities to involve your kids in the kitchen:

- **Recipe Selection:** Let your children help choose recipes from this cookbook. Involving them in the decision-making process makes them more excited to participate in the preparation.
- **Ingredient Prep:** Allow kids to wash fruits, measure ingredients, and mix mixtures. This hands-on involvement fosters confidence and a sense of accomplishment.
- **Creative Presentation:** Encourage kids to get creative with the presentation of dishes. They can help arrange toppings on smoothie bowls or decorate popsicles, making healthy eating more fun.
- **Theme Nights:** Host themed cooking nights where each family member can choose a cuisine or type of treat to prepare together. This not only encourages creativity but also exposes kids to different cultures and flavors.

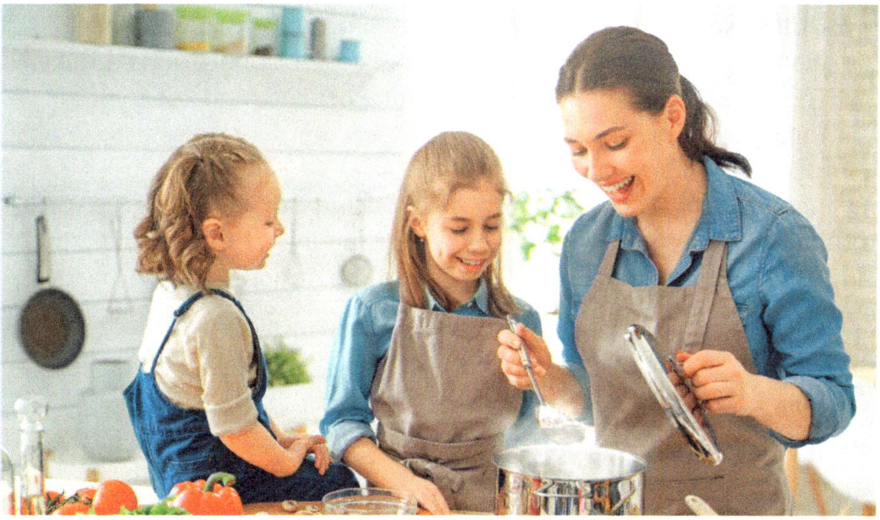

Staying Inspired

Resources and Support

Maintaining motivation can sometimes be a challenge, especially when trying to stick to a healthy eating plan. Here are some resources and strategies to keep you inspired:

1. **Follow Healthy Cooking Blogs and Influencers:** Stay connected with the vibrant community of health-focused bloggers and social media influencers. They often share new recipes, tips, and meal prep ideas that can inspire your culinary adventures.
2. **Join Cooking Classes:** Participating in local or online cooking classes focused on healthy recipes can provide new techniques and ideas while connecting you with like-minded individuals.
3. **Create a Recipe Journal:** Keep a journal of your favorite recipes, notes on what worked well, and ideas for future meals. This can serve as a great reference and help you stay organized in your meal planning.
4. **Engage with Your Community:** Attend local farmers' markets, health fairs, or cooking demonstrations in your area. These events can provide new ideas and introduce you to fresh, seasonal ingredients.
5. **Utilize Apps and Online Tools:** Many apps can help with meal planning, grocery shopping, and tracking your nutritional intake. These tools can simplify your cooking process and keep you focused on your health goals.

By incorporating these tips into your routine, you can navigate social situations with confidence, involve your family in the joy of cooking, and stay inspired in your journey toward healthier eating.

WHEN AND HOW TO USE PROTEIN SHAKES

Best Times to Consume Protein Shakes for Maximum Benefits

Protein shakes are a convenient and effective way to boost your protein intake, and there are specific times when consuming them can yield the best results. Here are some optimal moments to enjoy your protein shakes:

- **Post-Workout:** One of the most beneficial times to consume a protein shake is within 30 minutes after your workout. This period, often referred to as the "anabolic window," is crucial for muscle recovery and growth. A protein shake provides your body with the essential amino acids it needs to repair and build muscle tissue, helping to enhance recovery and performance.

- **Breakfast Replacement:** If you're pressed for time in the mornings, a protein shake can serve as a quick and nutritious breakfast option. Combining protein with fruits and healthy fats in a shake can keep you satiated and energized throughout the morning.

- **Mid-Afternoon Snack:** When the afternoon slump hits, a protein shake can help curb hunger and provide a sustained energy boost. It's an excellent way to avoid unhealthy snacking and keep your energy levels up until dinner.

- **Meal Supplement:** If you find it challenging to meet your protein goals through whole foods alone, consider using protein shakes as a supplement to your regular meals. They can be especially helpful for those on restricted diets or who have higher protein requirements due to fitness goals.

- **Before Bed:** Some individuals benefit from consuming a protein shake before bed, particularly if they are looking to support muscle recovery overnight. Casein protein, in particular, is known for its slow digestion rate, providing a steady release of amino acids throughout the night.

Tips for Incorporating Protein Shakes into an Active Lifestyle

Incorporating protein shakes into your daily routine can be a seamless process when you keep a few key strategies in mind:

- **Prep in Advance:** Prepare your protein shake ingredients in advance by portioning them into bags or containers. This makes it easy to blend a shake quickly when you're on the go. Pre-portioning fruits, greens, and protein powder can save you time and encourage you to stick to your healthy eating habits.
- **Experiment with Flavors:** Don't hesitate to mix and match different fruits, nut butters, and flavorings to keep your protein shakes exciting. Adding ingredients like spinach, kale, or even spices like cinnamon can enhance the nutritional value without compromising taste.
- **Stay Hydrated:** Remember to drink plenty of water throughout the day, especially if you're consuming protein shakes regularly. Staying hydrated is essential for overall health and can improve your performance during workouts.
- **Pair with Whole Foods:** For a balanced meal or snack, consider pairing your protein shake with whole foods. Enjoy it alongside a piece of fruit, a handful of nuts, or whole-grain toast for added fiber and nutrients.
- **Use as a Meal Replacement:** On particularly busy days, protein shakes can serve as meal replacements. However, ensure that they are well-balanced with carbohydrates and fats to create a complete meal. Including ingredients like oats or nut butter can help achieve this balance.
- **Listen to Your Body:** Pay attention to how your body responds to protein shakes. If you find certain ingredients are difficult to digest, adjust your recipes accordingly. Everyone's digestive system is different, and finding what works best for you is key.

HOW TO PREPARE ICE CREAM FOR ACTIVE LIFESTYLES

Quick Preparation Tips for Easy Consumption

When you lead an active lifestyle, having convenient and nutritious options on hand is essential. Preparing ice cream with the Ninja Creami can be a simple process, but there are a few tips you can follow to ensure that your frozen treats are ready for easy consumption:

- **Batch Prep in Advance:** Dedicate some time each week to prepare larger quantities of your favorite ice cream bases. This will save you time during busy days and ensure you always have healthy treats ready to go. Freeze your bases in the Ninja Creami pint containers so they are ready for processing when you want them.
- **Use Airtight Containers:** After processing your ice cream, transfer any leftovers to airtight containers. This helps maintain freshness and prevents freezer burn, allowing you to enjoy your treats over a longer period without losing quality.
- **Proper Freezing:** Ensure your ice cream is fully frozen before attempting to scoop. Ideally, let it freeze for at least 24 hours after processing. If you find it too hard, let it sit at room temperature for a few minutes before scooping for easier serving.
- **Thawing Techniques:** If your ice cream becomes too hard, simply run warm water over the outside of the pint container for a few seconds or let it sit out for 5-10 minutes. This will soften it enough for easy scooping.
- **Serving Sizes:** Consider portioning your ice cream into single-serving containers or cups. This makes it easy to grab a healthy treat on the go without the risk of overindulging.

Portable Protein Treats
for On-the-Go Nutrition

Incorporating protein-rich frozen treats into your busy lifestyle is a fantastic way to maintain energy levels and support recovery. Here are some ideas for portable protein treats that you can easily take with you:

1. **Protein Popsicles:** Use your Ninja Creami to create protein-packed popsicles that are easy to transport. Simply pour your favorite smoothie or protein shake mixture into popsicle molds, freeze, and enjoy a refreshing treat that's full of nutrients.

2. **Protein Energy Bites:** Prepare no-bake protein energy bites that can be stored in the fridge or freezer. These nutrient-dense bites are perfect for a quick snack and can be made with ingredients like oats, nut butters, and protein powder.

3. **Protein Bars:** Consider making homemade protein bars using your favorite protein powder, oats, and nut butter. Cut them into individual portions and store them in an airtight container for a convenient on-the-go snack.

4. **Portable Smoothie Jars:** Prepare smoothie jars the night before, filling jars with layers of fruits, yogurt, and protein powder. In the morning, just blend and enjoy! This option is both nutritious and easy to carry, making it perfect for busy mornings.

5. **Frozen Yogurt Bark:** Create a batch of frozen yogurt bark by spreading yogurt on a baking sheet and topping it with fruits, nuts, and seeds. Once frozen, break it into pieces and store them in a container for a quick, nutritious snack.

Recommended Healthy Cooking Blogs and Influencers

Staying inspired in the kitchen is essential for maintaining a healthy lifestyle. Here are some of my favorite healthy cooking blogs and influencers that provide a wealth of resources, recipes, and tips for nutritious eating:

1. **minimalistbaker.com:** This blog focuses on simple, quick recipes that require 10 ingredients or less, are easily accessible, and are often plant-based. It's a fantastic resource for those looking to simplify their cooking without sacrificing flavor.
2. **ohsheglows.com:** This award-winning blog features a variety of wholesome, plant-based recipes that are both nourishing and delicious. Angela Liddon, the creator, shares personal stories and tips for healthy living that resonate with many readers.
3. **fitfoodiefinds.com:** A great source for healthy recipes that don't skimp on flavor, this blog offers a wide variety of meal ideas, meal prep tips, and fitness inspiration to help you stay on track with your health goals.
4. **nutritionstripped.com:** Run by registered dietitian McKel Kooienga, this blog focuses on whole foods and balanced nutrition. It offers a wealth of resources, including meal plans, recipes, and wellness tips that are rooted in science.
5. **thehealthymaven.com:** This blog provides a mix of healthy recipes, wellness tips, and lifestyle content. Davina's approachable style encourages readers to embrace healthy eating without feeling deprived.

Celebrating Healthy Eating
with the Ninja Creami

As we wrap up **Nutritionist's Ninja Creami Protein Cookbook Recipes 2025**, I want to take a moment to reflect on the journey we've shared in exploring the world of homemade frozen treats. The Ninja Creami is not just an appliance; it's a gateway to a healthier lifestyle, allowing you to create delightful desserts that satisfy your cravings while providing nourishment. By embracing the recipes in this cookbook, you are taking important steps toward making healthy eating enjoyable and accessible for you and your family.

Each recipe has been crafted with care, focusing on wholesome ingredients that bring joy and satisfaction without compromising your health goals. From rich chocolate ice creams to refreshing fruit sorbets, the possibilities are endless. I encourage you to use this cookbook as a springboard for creativity in your kitchen. Don't hesitate to experiment with flavors, textures, and ingredients to develop your unique frozen treats that reflect your tastes and nutritional needs.

Thank You and Encouragement for Your Culinary Journey

Thank you for choosing The Unofficial CHEFMAN Air Fryer Cookbook for Quick & Healthy Week Nights as your guide to healthier cooking. I hope this book has inspired you to embrace the art of cooking and has equipped you with the tools and recipes needed to create delicious meals for yourself and your loved ones.

As you embark on your culinary journey, remember that every meal is an opportunity to nourish your body and share love with those around you. Cooking is a skill that can be refined over time, so don't be discouraged by challenges or mishaps in the kitchen. Each experience is a chance to learn and grow.

I encourage you to keep exploring new flavors, experiment with ingredients, and share your culinary creations with family and friends. Engage with your community, whether it's through cooking classes, social media, or local food events. The more you connect with others who share your passion for healthy eating, the more motivated you'll become.

Lastly, always prioritize your well-being. Listen to your body, enjoy the foods you love, and make choices that support your health goals. With the CHEFMAN Air Fryer, you have a powerful tool at your disposal to create meals that are not only nutritious but also enjoyable.

Here's to your continued success in the kitchen and to many delicious, healthy meals ahead!

Hi There!

I hope you are enjoying my book so far. I would really appreciate it if you could leave a quick review on Amazon.

Just simply scan the code below using your mobile phone's camera, or you can enter the link below on our web browser.

https://swiy.com/ReviewCreami3

Thanks a lot!

- Clara

INDEX

The Index is designed to help you quickly locate specific recipes, ingredients, and topics within The Nutritionist's Ninja Creami Healthy Recipes Cookbook 2025: Healthy Guilt-Free Treats with Nutritious Ingredients. Whether you're searching for a particular frozen treat, looking for recipes that fit dietary restrictions, or exploring various ingredient options, this index will guide you efficiently to what you need.

Made in the USA
Monee, IL
03 November 2026

67384559R00049